HUMAN PAPILLOMAVIRUS

(HPV)

I0446848

Unlocking the Secrets of HPV:

Your Roadmap to Health and

Empowerment

BY

Dr. Luna Jefferson

Copyright

TABLE OF CONTENT

INTRODUCTION

Explaining the Importance of the Topic

The subject of Human Papilloma infection (HPV) and its related medical problems is of fundamental significance for a few convincing reasons. Its importance rises above clinical limits, including cultural, profound, and general wellbeing aspects. Here are a few key perspectives that underline the essential significance of this point:

1. Widespread Prevalence: HPV is one of the most well-known physically communicated diseases around the world. The sheer predominance of this infection implies that countless people, particularly the more youthful age, are in danger of contracting

it. Understanding HPV is indispensable for individual wellbeing and public prosperity.

2. Connection to Cancer: Certain high-risk HPV strains are connected to different diseases, most strikingly cervical malignant growth. Cervical malignant growth, however exceptionally preventable and treatable when identified early, stays one of the main sources of disease related passings among ladies universally. Information on HPV and its part in malignant growth is urgent for avoidance and early discovery.

3. Prevention Through Vaccination: HPV vaccinations have been created and demonstrated powerful in forestalling the infection and related diseases. Understanding the significance of inoculation and advancing it is a key general wellbeing drive, with the possibility to save incalculable lives.

4. Emotional and Social Impact: HPV can socially affect people and their families. Shame, dread, and deception are normal difficulties. By tending to these viewpoints, the subject becomes significant restoratively as well as genuinely and culturally.

5. General Wellbeing Advocacy: Upholding for HPV mindfulness, vaccinations, and further developed admittance to medical services assets can impact general wellbeing approaches and diminish the weight of HPV-related sicknesses. Individual and aggregate backing endeavors are fundamental.

In summary, the significance of HPV and its related medical problems lies in its predominance, its connect to malignant growth, the accessibility of anticipation through vaccination, the close to home and social effect it conveys, and the potential for general wellbeing backing. By getting it and tending to this theme, we move toward a better future for all.

Sharing the Purpose of the Book

The purpose of this book is multi-layered, driven by a promise to information, mindfulness, and strengthening. Its center mission is to give a far reaching asset that fills a few basic needs:

1. Education and Awareness: The book aims to instruct readers about Human Papilloma infection (HPV) and its related medical problems, offering a balanced comprehension of this common

yet frequently misread infection. It enlightens the logical perspectives, transmission, counteraction, and ramifications of HPV, engaging people with the information they need to come to informed conclusions about their wellbeing.

2. Prevention and Advocacy: A focal reason for the book is to advocate for HPV anticipation. By revealing insight into the significance of vaccination, ordinary screenings, and safe sex rehearses, it urges perusers to find proactive ways to shield themselves as well as other people from the infection and its potential wellbeing gambles.

3. Profound and Viable Support: Past clinical information, this book stretches out a strong hand to those impacted by HPV-related medical problems. It offers direction on adapting to the profound perspectives and useful difficulties of living with HPV, encouraging flexibility and strengthening.

4. Engaging Advocacy: The book calls readers to become advocates for HPV mindfulness and general wellbeing. It furnishes them with the data and inspiration to impact strategy changes, dissipate legends and confusions, and join the development to lessen the weight of HPV-related sicknesses.

5. Community Building: This book means to make a feeling of local area among people exploring HPV-related difficulties. It shares accounts of strength, cultivates a feeling of having a place, and urges perusers to interface and backing each other.

Basically, the reason for this book is to be a directing light through the frequently perplexing and vilified universe of HPV. It tries to engage people with information, motivate backing, offer close to home and functional help, and at last add to a future where HPV-related sicknesses are limited, and the prosperity of everything is upgraded.

CHAPTER ONE

Unmasking the Hidden Threat

In a world filled with clinical secrets, Human Papillomavirus, or HPV, remains as a secret danger influencing a great many lives. This part strips back the cover of mystery encompassing this normal yet frequently misconstrued infection, revealing insight into its predominance and effect.

HPV is a confounding substance, famous for its secretive attack of the human body. Unbeknownst to many, it is the most pervasive physically communicated disease around the world. This unavoidable infection, described by a bunch of strains, can influence all kinds of people, youthful and old. Notwithstanding its commonness, most of those tainted stay ignorant about its presence because of its generally expected asymptomatic nature.

The Mysterious World of HPV

To genuinely get a handle on the meaning of Human Papillomavirus (HPV), it is basic to understand its commonness and the significant effect it uses on the worldwide scene of general wellbeing. This section dives into the surprising insights and broad ramifications of this inescapable and frequently quiet popular presence.

HPV's pervasiveness is faltering. It is the most considered normal physically communicated disease around the world. A large number of people, paying little heed to mature, race, or orientation, end up contacted by its presence. As a matter of fact, it's assessed that a critical level of physically dynamic individuals will experience HPV sooner or later in their lives. This omnipresence rises above borders, making HPV a worldwide wellbeing concern.

Why Every Individual Should Be Aware

In a world loaded up with wellbeing concerns and clinical complexities, the awareness of Human Papillomavirus, or HPV, remains as a foremost need. This part highlights the convincing justifications for why each person, paying little heed to mature, orientation, or foundation, ought to be very much in the know about the presence and potential dangers related with HPV.

HPV, most importantly, is pervasive, making it an issue that rises above boundaries and socioeconomics. It's one of the most well-known physically sent contaminations internationally, with the possibility to influence practically any individual who is physically dynamic. The universality of HPV is a convincing motivation to be careful, as nobody is really invulnerable to its scope.

Also, the potential wellbeing chances related with HPV, especially the high-risk strains, are not to be undervalued. Cervical disease, among different malignancies, is an impressive foe that frequently emerges from untreated HPV contaminations. Monitoring this association is urgent, as it stresses the significance of early location, inoculation, and preventive measures.

Besides, understanding HPV encourages a feeling of strengthening. Information prepares people to arrive at informed conclusions about their sexual wellbeing, make fitting preventive moves, and participate in open discussions with medical care suppliers. It destroys the cover of obliviousness that can sustain the spread of this infection.

Finally, HPV mindfulness isn't restricted to individual wellbeing; it reaches out to general wellbeing. By staying alert and proactive, people add to the aggregate exertion of diminishing HPV-related sicknesses, at last pursuing a better society. In this shared mindset lies the solidarity to handle the secret danger that is HPV, guaranteeing a more splendid and better future for all.

CHAPTER TWO

The HPV Puzzle: Types and Transmission

Grasping Human Papilloma infection (HPV) requires unwinding a mind boggling puzzle made out of a variety of viral kinds and many-sided transmission pathways. This part enlightens the variety of HPV strains and the components through which it tracks down its direction into our lives.

HPV is definitely not a solid substance; it's a mosaic of more than 200 extraordinary sorts, each with its own qualities and inclinations. Some are classified as okay, causing harmless skin moles or genital moles, while others are assigned high-risk because of their capability to prompt malignant growth. This variety adds layers of unpredictability to the HPV puzzle, as the infection's different signs and wellbeing suggestions request intensive comprehension.

Transmission is the second piece of the riddle. HPV doesn't stick to a solitary course of disease; it's sent through skin-to-skin contact, particularly through sexual action. The infection, covered in its puzzling imperceptibility, can be moved easily. This mind boggling method of transmission, including everything from sex to non-sexual touch, highlights the need of mindfulness and preventive measures.

As we explore the maze of HPV types and unwind the strings of transmission, it becomes clear that this puzzle isn't simply a scholarly activity. It's a critical excursion towards perceiving the extent of HPV's effect on our lives. Equipped with this information, we can settle on informed conclusions about our sexual wellbeing and, simultaneously, shield ourselves from the perplexing trap of HPV contaminations.

Demystifying the Different HPV Strains

The universe of Human Papilloma infection (HPV) isn't solid however an embroidery of variety, holding onto more than 200 distinct strains. In this section, we leave on an excursion to demystify the complexities of these HPV strains, uncovering the changing jobs they play in human wellbeing and the results they can bring.

HPV strains fall into two principal classifications: okay and high-risk. Generally safe strains are liable for the infamous moles that show up on the skin or private parts, causing uneasiness and restorative worries. These strains are by and large harmless and may precipitously clear without mediation. Notwithstanding, the high-risk strains possess a really threatening spot in the HPV scene. These strains are related with a range of malignant growths, including cervical, butt-centric, and oropharyngeal disease. Their presence fills in as an obvious sign of HPV's capability to cause extreme, life changing outcomes.

As we disentangle the different HPV strains, it becomes apparent that every one has special qualities, ways of behaving, and suggestions for wellbeing. This information is essential, as it fills in as the establishment whereupon informed choices can be made. Whether it's embracing vaccination, rehearsing safe sex, or grasping the dangers of specific strains, demystifying the variety of HPV strains enables people to safeguard their prosperity. In this part, we step into the universe of HPV types, prepared to face its intricacy and go with informed decisions for a better future.

How HPV Spreads: From Skin to Closeness

Grasping how Human Papilloma infection (HPV) spreads is fundamental to demystifying this unavoidable infection. This part enlightens the perplexing pathways through which HPV ventures, from easygoing contact to imply collaborations.

HPV is an expert of mask, fit for invading the body through various courses. One of the most well-known is skin-to-skin contact. This can incorporate anything from a basic handshake to insinuate connections. The infection can be tracked down on the skin, including the genital and butt-centric regions, and can undoubtedly move starting with one individual then onto the next. This reality highlights the meaning of safe sex rehearses, as even apparently innocuous actual contact can prompt transmission.

Sexual closeness is an essential method of transmission. HPV is frequently alluded to as a physically communicated contamination since it flourishes in the genital and butt-centric locales. Whether through vaginal, butt-centric, or oral sex, the infection can be passed starting with one accomplice then onto the next. Condoms give some insurance yet don't dispense with the gamble altogether, as HPV can taint regions not covered by the hindrance.

The transmission of HPV isn't exclusively restricted to sexual accomplices. It tends to be gone through non-sexual contact too, for example, during labor or through close skin-to-skin contact in settings like storage spaces or shared towels.

As we venture through the complexities of HPV transmission, obviously cautiousness and understanding are our most noteworthy partners. Information engages people to pursue informed decisions about their sexual wellbeing and, simultaneously, lessen the gamble of HPV transmission. This section focuses a light on the pathways through which HPV spreads, underlining the significance of safe practices and mindfulness.

The Hidden Dangers of Common Behaviors

In our everyday lives, seemingly innocuous behaviors can unwittingly expose us to the hidden dangers of Human Papilloma virus (HPV). This chapter uncovers how routine activities can inadvertently facilitate the transmission of HPV and contribute to the virus's prevalence.

One common behavior that often goes unnoticed is simple physical contact. A handshake, a hug, or sharing towels may seem harmless, but these actions can transmit HPV. The virus resides on the skin, making it easily transferable through close contact. This hidden danger emphasizes the importance of maintaining good hygiene and considering the potential risks associated with shared items.

Another often underestimated behavior is the act of oral sex. Many are unaware that HPV can be transmitted through this form of sexual intimacy. The throat, just like the genital and anal areas, can harbor the virus, raising the risk of oropharyngeal cancers. This hidden danger underscores the need for comprehensive sexual education and safe sex practices.

Furthermore, ignoring regular check-ups and screenings is a common behavior that can have severe consequences. Cervical cancer, strongly linked to HPV, can be prevented or detected early through routine screenings. By neglecting these check-ups, individuals unknowingly increase their risk of HPV-related health issues.

This chapter urges us to be mindful of these hidden dangers and consider the implications of seemingly ordinary behaviors. By doing so, we can take steps to protect our health, embrace safe practices, and ultimately reduce the impact of HPV on our lives. It underscores the importance of education and awareness to empower individuals in navigating the potential risks of common behaviors.

CHAPTER THREE

Guarding Against HPV: Your Shield of Prevention

In the continuous fight against Human Papilloma infection (HPV), prevention remains as the most powerful weapon in our stockpile. This section digs into the different techniques accessible to people, offering them a vigorous safeguard to prepare for HPV and its possible results.

Vaccination, first and foremost, is the foundation of prevention. HPV antibodies, like Gardasil and Cervarix, have arisen as strong partners. They have the ability to safeguard against the most widely recognized high-risk HPV types answerable for diseases and okay sorts causing moles. This part unloads the security and viability of antibodies, destroys misinterpretations, and highlights the meaning of vaccination in ruining HPV's effect.

Safe sex rehearses arise as one more necessary part of HPV avoidance. Condoms, while not secure, can lessen the gamble of transmission during sexual contact. Exhaustive sexual training and correspondence with accomplices become fundamental apparatuses in the fight against HPV's sexual transmission.

Schooling about the infection and its suggestions is likewise an imperative piece of the counteraction safeguard. Mindfulness engages people to arrive at informed conclusions about their sexual wellbeing, supports normal check-ups, and prompts ideal intercessions.

This part supports the significance of counteraction as a powerful safeguard against HPV. Whether through vaccination, safe sex practices, or schooling, people possess the ability to shield themselves from the infection's secretive interruption. By using this safeguard of anticipation, they assume command over their wellbeing and add to the more extensive work to diminish the weight of HPV-related infections.

Uncovering the Force of Counteraction

Counteraction isn't simply an idea; a strong power can shape the course of general wellbeing. With regards to Human Papilloma infection (HPV), disclosing the force of avoidance is vital in deflecting the dangers and results related with this normal yet frequently underrated infection.

At the very front of HPV counteraction is vaccination. HPV vaccinations have demonstrated to be profoundly successful in protecting people from the most harmful strains, lessening the gamble of different malignant growths. The force of these antibodies lies in their capacity to intrude on the infection's transmission at its source, giving dependable security.

Instruction arises as one more powerful mainstay of avoidance. It furnishes people with the information expected to come to informed conclusions about their sexual wellbeing, consequently empowering them to safeguard themselves and their accomplices. Informed decisions lessen the gamble of HPV transmission and the potential for unexpected problems.

Safe sex rehearses total the trifecta of counteraction. Condoms, while not faultless, go about as a hindrance against HPV during sexual contact, further lessening the gamble of disease. Joining safe sex rehearses with vaccination and training structures a vigorous guard against the infection's spread.

Divulging the force of counteraction is an enabling excursion that at last permits people to assume command over their wellbeing. By embracing vaccination, schooling, and safe practices, we make a defensive safeguard against HPV's covert interruption. This section enlightens the strength of avoidance and the significant effect it can have on people and general wellbeing at large.

Vaccination: Your Ultimate Weapon

In the fight against Human Papilloma virus (HPV), vaccination stands as the ultimate weapon, a formidable shield that can protect individuals from the most common high-risk HPV types, reducing the risk of several cancers. This chapter unveils the power of vaccination, highlighting its safety, efficacy, and the profound impact it has on personal and public health.

HPV vaccines, such as Gardasil and Cervarix, have proven their mettle in preventing infection with the most troublesome HPV strains. They offer robust protection, effectively reducing the risk of cervical, anal, and oropharyngeal cancers. The safety of these vaccines is well-established, with extensive research and real-world evidence demonstrating their minimal side effects.

One of the key misconceptions about HPV vaccines is that they are solely for women. This chapter dispels this myth, emphasizing that vaccination is equally important for men. By vaccinating both genders, we create a powerful collective defense against HPV, reducing its transmission within the population.

Moreover, vaccination can be a lifesaver when administered early. The recommended age for HPV vaccination is ideally before sexual activity begins, as this is when the vaccine is most effective. However, it's never too late to get vaccinated, as it can still provide valuable protection.

In unveiling the power of vaccination, this chapter underscores that it is not just a personal choice; it is a community and public health imperative. By embracing vaccination, individuals fortify themselves against the insidious threat of HPV and contribute to a healthier, HPV-protected future for all.

Safe Sex Secrets: Reducing Your Risk

Safe sex is an integral component of the arsenal against Human Papilloma virus (HPV). This chapter unveils the "safe sex secrets," a set of practices and principles that empower individuals to reduce their risk of HPV infection and its potentially life-altering consequences.

Condoms, often regarded as the unsung heroes of safe sex, play a pivotal role in reducing the risk of HPV transmission during sexual activity. These barrier methods, while not foolproof, act as a protective shield, creating a physical barrier between partners that can significantly reduce the chance of HPV transmission. Using condoms consistently and correctly is key to their effectiveness.

Open communication with sexual partners is another crucial "safe sex secret." Discussing sexual histories, previous HPV vaccinations, and health concerns helps build trust and understanding between partners. This dialogue can lead to informed decisions about sexual activity, protecting both individuals from HPV and other sexually transmitted infections. Comprehensive sexual education is a fundamental aspect of reducing HPV risk. By understanding the modes of transmission and the potential consequences of HPV, individuals are better equipped to make informed choices about their sexual health. Encouraging routine check-ups and screenings can also lead to early detection and intervention.

By delving into these "safe sex secrets," this chapter empowers individuals to take charge of their sexual health and reduce their risk of HPV infection. Safe sex practices, combined with vaccination and education, form a comprehensive defense against the virus, ensuring a healthier and more informed approach to sexual relationships and well-being.

CHAPTER FOUR

The Ticking Time Bomb: HPV and Health Risks

Human Papilloma virus (HPV) is often referred to as a ticking time bomb, quietly lurking within individuals and potentially setting the stage for serious health risks. This chapter delves into the latent dangers of HPV, its association with various health issues, and the imperative for early detection and prevention.

HPV infections, particularly the high-risk strains, are like a hidden menace. They can persist in the body, often asymptomatic and unnoticed, for years or even decades. During this silent period, they can gradually induce changes in the affected tissues, setting the stage for the development of cancers, most notably cervical, anal, and oropharyngeal cancers.

Cervical cancer is perhaps the most prominent and devastating consequence of persistent high-risk HPV infections. It serves as a grim reminder of the potential health risks associated with the virus. Routine screenings, such as Pap smears and HPV tests, are critical for early detection and intervention, helping to defuse the ticking time bomb before it detonates.

The chapter also explores the psychological and emotional impact of an HPV diagnosis, revealing the fear and anxiety it can evoke. By shedding light on the potential health risks and the emotional toll of HPV, this chapter underscores the urgency of proactive measures, including vaccination and regular screenings, in preventing the time bomb of HPV from wreaking havoc on lives. Ultimately, it advocates for vigilance and early action to mitigate the health risks associated with this silent and potentially destructive virus.

The Silent Culprit Behind Serious Health Issues

Human Papilloma virus (HPV) is a silent, insidious culprit that often operates unnoticed, yet it is responsible for a range of serious health issues. This chapter peels back the layers of HPV's stealthy invasion and its association with various health complications, underscoring the importance of awareness and proactive measures.

HPV's inconspicuous nature is its hallmark. Many individuals carry the virus unknowingly, as it frequently remains asymptomatic. This invisibility allows it to establish a presence in the body, gradually increasing the risk of health problems, particularly when high-risk strains are involved.

One of the most alarming health issues linked to HPV is cervical cancer. It is a dire consequence of persistent high-risk HPV infections and serves as a poignant illustration of the virus's sinister potential. Yet, this silent culprit extends its reach to other cancers, including those of the anus, penis, throat, and more. These conditions often emerge years after the initial HPV infection, making early detection a vital defense.

This chapter also delves into the emotional and psychological toll of an HPV diagnosis. The fear and uncertainty it brings to individuals' lives can be just as debilitating as the physical consequences. By unveiling HPV's silent role in these serious health issues, the chapter emphasizes the necessity of prevention through vaccination and regular screenings. It urges individuals to shatter the silence and take control of their health, refusing to let the stealthy invader hold sway over their lives.

The Journey from Infection to Cancer

The journey from Human Papilloma virus (HPV) infection to cancer is a complex and perilous path that highlights the profound impact of this insidious virus. This chapter traces this journey, emphasizing the importance of understanding the stages and taking proactive measures to disrupt it.

HPV infection often begins innocuously, with the virus entering the body through sexual contact or other modes of transmission. In many cases, it remains dormant, with no noticeable symptoms. However, if high-risk HPV strains are present, the virus can infiltrate cells in the genital or oropharyngeal areas, and the journey toward cancer begins.

The journey consists of several stages. Initially, the virus can cause cellular changes, which might lead to the development of genital warts. But for those infected with high-risk HPV types, the situation can escalate. Persistent infection can lead to the transformation of normal cells into precancerous lesions. If left unchecked, these precancerous cells may further evolve into full-blown cancer.

Cervical cancer is one of the most well-documented consequences of persistent high-risk HPV infection. This journey is marked by gradual changes in cervical cells that can ultimately culminate in invasive cancer, often years after the initial infection.

Understanding this journey is critical as it underscores the importance of early detection and intervention. Regular screenings, such as Pap smears and HPV tests, are vital checkpoints along this path. By monitoring for signs of cellular changes, healthcare professionals can take action to prevent the progression to cancer, disrupting the perilous journey from infection to malignancy.

Early Detection: The Lifesaving Key

In the realm of Human Papillomavirus (HPV), early detection emerges as the vital key to saving lives and preventing the progression of potentially devastating health issues. This chapter underscores the profound significance of timely screenings, monitoring, and intervention in the face of HPV's silent and often sinister threat.

HPV is often a stealthy invader, capable of lingering in the body for years without any noticeable symptoms. During this silent phase, the virus can cause subtle yet crucial cellular changes that may evolve into precancerous or cancerous conditions. Early detection acts as a sentinel, a mechanism for spotting these subtle transformations before they become life-threatening.

Routine screenings, such as Pap smears and HPV tests, are the primary tools for early detection. These tests are essential in monitoring the health of the cervix and identifying any cellular abnormalities. When identified early, these abnormalities can be managed and treated before they have a chance to progress into cancer.

Cervical cancer, one of the most closely associated health risks with HPV, serves as a poignant example of the importance of early detection. This cancer, often the result of persistent high-risk HPV infection, can be prevented or detected at an early, highly treatable stage through screenings.

This chapter aims to shine a spotlight on the transformative power of early detection. By conducting regular screenings and heeding the early warning signs, individuals can take control of their health and ensure that HPV's potential health risks are defused before they have a chance to reach a critical stage. Early detection is indeed the lifesaving key that can protect individuals from the insidious impact of HPV.

CHAPTER FIVE

Vaccination: Your Armor of Protection

In the tireless fight against Human Papilloma infection (HPV), vaccination fills in as the secure reinforcement of security, making preparations for an unavoidable and possibly obliterating enemy. This part reveals the groundbreaking force of vaccination, clarifying its wellbeing, viability, and its fantastic job in safeguarding people from HPV-related wellbeing gambles.

HPV antibodies, like Gardasil and Cervarix, have arisen as genuine sentinels, equipped for bracing the human body against the most deceptive kinds of the infection. They have gone through thorough testing and have demonstrated to be protected as well as exceptionally compelling. These vaccinations give far reaching insurance against the most well-known high-risk HPV types, which are liable for different tumors.

The way in to the vaccinations' viability lies in their capacity to get a powerful safe reaction. When directed, they animate the development of antibodies, preparing the invulnerable framework to perceive and battle the infection whenever experienced. This proactive safeguard system keeps contamination from flourishing, fundamentally diminishing the gamble of HPV-related infections.

Dispersing normal confusions, this section accentuates that HPV inoculation isn't restricted to one orientation. It is fundamental for the two guys and females, as HPV influences everybody. By inoculating all, we make an aggregate safeguard against the infection, lessening its transmission inside the populace and at last decreasing its effect on general wellbeing.

In divulging the force of vaccination, this part features that it isn't simply an individual decision; it is a local area and general wellbeing basic. By embracing vaccination, people wear this shield of security, guaranteeing a better and safer future despite HPV's expected dangers.

The HPV vaccination: Demonstrated Wellbeing and Adequacy

In the fight against Human Papilloma infection (HPV), vaccinations are our considerable partners, offering demonstrated wellbeing and viability in forestalling HPV-related wellbeing chances. This part reveals the science and security behind HPV antibodies, accentuating their basic job in shielding people from this normal yet possibly life changing infection.

HPV antibodies, including Gardasil and Cervarix, have gone through thorough testing and have demonstrated to be astoundingly protected and powerful. Clinical preliminaries including large number of members have exhibited their ability to safeguard against the most widely recognized high-risk HPV types liable for diseases, including cervical, butt-centric, and oropharyngeal tumors.

Wellbeing is foremost in vaccination improvement, and the HPV antibodies are no exemption. Broad checking has affirmed their wellbeing, with revealed aftereffects being by and large gentle, for example, torment at the infusion site or gentle fever. Serious unfriendly impacts are really interesting, accentuating the antibodies' solid security profile.

The vaccinations' viability lies in their capacity to invigorate a strong safe reaction. Upon vaccination, the body produces antibodies that can perceive and ward off the infection whenever uncovered from now on. This insusceptibility keeps the infection from laying out contamination, consequently lessening the gamble of HPV-related sicknesses.

Exposing fantasies and misguided judgments, this section confirms that HPV inoculation is a protected, viable, and life-saving measure. It highlights the vaccinations' job in diminishing the weight of HPV-related wellbeing gambles and the critical commitment they make to general wellbeing. By revealing the science and security behind HPV vaccinations, this section engages people to go with informed decisions and embrace inoculation as a safeguard against HPV's possible dangers.

Debunking Myths and Misconceptions

In the realm of Human Papilloma virus (HPV), myths and misconceptions often overshadow the facts, hindering awareness, prevention, and early intervention. This section dives into the most prevalent misconceptions about HPV, unraveling the truths that dispel the fog of misinformation and empower individuals to make informed decisions.

One of the most pervasive myths is that HPV affects only women. In reality, HPV is an equal-opportunity virus, impacting both men and women. Men can contract and transmit the virus just as easily as women, and they are also at risk of developing HPV-related health issues. Debunking this myth underscores the importance of HPV vaccination for both genders.

Another common misconception is that HPV vaccines promote risky sexual behavior. The truth is that these vaccines protect against a virus with serious health risks, making them an important tool for preventive healthcare. They do not encourage riskier behavior but instead provide protection against an invisible threat.

Additionally, concerns about vaccine safety often arise. Extensive research and real-world evidence support the safety of HPV vaccines. Serious adverse effects are exceedingly rare, while the benefits of vaccination in reducing the risk of cancer far outweigh any potential risks.

By addressing these myths and misconceptions, this chapter empowers individuals to navigate the complexities of HPV with accurate information. In debunking these fallacies, it highlights the importance of evidence-based knowledge, encouraging people to embrace vaccination, engage in safe sex practices, and pursue regular screenings to protect their health and well-being.

Empowering Yourself Through Vaccination

In the ongoing battle against Human Papilloma virus (HPV), vaccination emerges as a potent tool of empowerment. This chapter underscores the transformative power of vaccination in equipping individuals to take control of their health, reduce their HPV risk, and contribute to a future free from the burden of HPV-related diseases.

HPV vaccination is a pivotal aspect of preventive healthcare, offering individuals a proactive means of safeguarding their well-being. By receiving the vaccine, individuals empower themselves to build immunity against the most common high-risk HPV types responsible for various cancers, including cervical, anal, and oropharyngeal cancers. This proactive defense can significantly reduce the risk of infection and its potential consequences.

Vaccination is not only about personal protection but also community well-being. By embracing vaccination, individuals participate in a collective effort to create herd immunity, reducing the overall transmission of HPV within the population. This communal defense can eventually lead to the eradication of the virus and its associated health risks.

Debunking myths and misconceptions, this chapter emphasizes that HPV vaccination is not an endorsement of risky sexual behavior; rather, it is a vital tool for preventive healthcare. It encourages individuals, both young and old, to explore the transformative power of vaccination and take the steps necessary to protect their health. By embracing vaccination, individuals not only empower themselves but also contribute to a healthier, HPV-protected future for all.

CHAPTER SIX

Diagnosis and Treatment: Navigating the Storm

With regards to Human Papilloma infection (HPV) and its related wellbeing gambles, the excursion doesn't end with mindfulness and anticipation — it reaches out to finding and treatment. This part investigates the difficulties and intricacies of exploring the tempest of HPV-related medical problems, from early identification to overseeing and treating the outcomes.

Conclusion starts with routine screenings, for example, Pap spreads and HPV tests, that intend to identify cell changes characteristic of HPV disease and likely precancerous or malignant circumstances. Early discovery is the principal help, offering people the opportunity to mediate and get treatment at a sensible stage.

At the point when HPV-related medical problems are analyzed, different therapies become possibly the most important factor.

These may incorporate surgeries, radiation treatment, or chemotherapy, contingent upon the seriousness and degree of the condition. The decision of therapy still up in the air by factors like the kind of disease, its stage, and the singular's general wellbeing.

In the tempest of determination and treatment, close to home and mental difficulties can be basically as overwhelming as the actual ones. A conclusion of a HPV-related condition can bring tension and dread. Emotionally supportive networks, including medical services experts and friends and family, are vital in assisting people with exploring these tempestuous waters.

This section enlightens the complexities of finding and therapy with regards to HPV, recognizing both the clinical and close to home parts of the excursion. It accentuates the significance of early location and mediation and offers trust by featuring the advances in clinical science that keep on working on the possibilities of recuperation. At last, it fills in as a directing light for those exploring the tempest of HPV-related medical problems, giving data and backing to assist people with settling on informed choices and assume command over their wellbeing.

The Critical point in time: HPV Finding

The critical point in time in the fight against Human Papilloma infection (HPV) frequently shows up with a finding. This part dives into the perplexing feelings and useful ramifications that go with a HPV determination, offering experiences on how people can explore this crucial second.

For some, a HPV conclusion comes after routine screenings, for example, Pap spreads and HPV tests. These tests can recognize the presence of the infection and distinguish cell changes in the cervix or other impacted regions. The insight about a HPV conclusion can be sincerely charged, igniting dread, disarray, and vulnerability.

Understanding the kind of HPV and its potential dangers is fundamental. Okay HPV types ordinarily cause moles, while high-risk types are related with the improvement of diseases. This information frames the establishment for informed choices about medical services and follow-up activities.

Exploring the tempest of a HPV finding frequently needs help. Medical services experts assume an essential part in directing people through the cycle, making sense of the ramifications of the determination, and suggesting proper therapy or observing. Basic encouragement from friends and family is similarly vital, giving a consoling presence during a period of pain.

This part fills in as a compass during the critical point in time, revealing insight into the intricacies of HPV finding and the personal difficulties it brings. It enables people to look for help, get clarification on some pressing issues, and arrive at informed conclusions about their medical services venture. By facing the critical point in time with mental fortitude and understanding, people can assume command over their wellbeing and, if vital, leave on a way to oversee and treat HPV-related medical problems.

A Road map for Treatment and Management

When an HPV-related diagnosis is confirmed, a road map for treatment and management becomes a lifeline, guiding individuals through the complex journey ahead. This chapter illuminates the key steps, decisions, and considerations that compose this road map, offering insights on how to navigate the challenges and uncertainties that HPV-related health issues can bring.

The road map begins with a clear understanding of the diagnosis, including the type of HPV, the extent of cellular changes, and the potential risks involved. This knowledge serves as the cornerstone for informed decisions about treatment options and the course of action to be taken.

Treatment choices can vary depending on the specific HPV-related health issue. Surgical procedures, radiation therapy, chemotherapy, or other interventions may be recommended. The decision is often influenced by factors such as the type and stage of cancer, the patient's overall health, and their preferences.

Support and communication are integral to this journey. Healthcare professionals play a central role in providing guidance and expertise. They can help individuals navigate the complexities of treatment options, side effects, and recovery. Emotional support from loved ones and support groups can also provide solace and encouragement during this challenging period.

The road map emphasizes the importance of taking an active role in one's healthcare journey. Asking questions, seeking second opinions, and staying informed are vital components. By following the road map for treatment and management, individuals can navigate the complexities of HPV-related health issues with resilience, hope, and a sense of control.

Insights from Survivors: Stories of Resilience

Amid the challenges posed by Human Papilloma virus (HPV) and its associated health issues, survivors' stories serve as beacons of hope and resilience. This chapter presents insights from survivors who have navigated the complexities of HPV-related diagnoses and treatments, offering inspiration and valuable lessons for others on a similar journey.

Survivors of HPV-related health issues often highlight the power of early detection and proactive healthcare. Many have stressed the importance of routine screenings, which allowed them to identify and address the condition at a manageable stage. These insights underscore the significance of regular medical check-ups in preventing or managing HPV-related diseases.

Furthermore, survivors emphasize the crucial role of emotional support from healthcare professionals, loved ones, and support networks. Their stories reveal that the journey is not just a physical one but a deeply emotional and psychological one. The strength to endure and persevere often comes from the understanding and compassion of others.

Survivors' stories also underscore the importance of maintaining a positive mindset and a sense of control. They emphasize the value of seeking information, asking questions, and being actively involved in treatment decisions. By sharing their experiences, they empower others to confront HPV-related health issues with determination and hope.

In weaving together these stories of resilience and triumph, this chapter provides valuable insights into the complexities of HPV-related health challenges. These survivors' journeys serve as testaments to the power of early detection, emotional support, and personal resilience. Their stories offer a source of inspiration and guidance for those navigating similar paths, proving that there is hope and strength to be found in the face of HPV-related health issues.

CHAPTER SEVEN

Rising Above the Challenge: Your Emotional Journey

In the domain of Human Papilloma infection (HPV) and its related medical problems, the close to home excursion is pretty much as critical as the actual one. This section investigates the significant inner difficulties that people face when gone up against with HPV, offering experiences on the most proficient method to explore this part of the excursion and arise more grounded.

A HPV conclusion frequently blends a scope of feelings, including dread, tension, disarray, and even disgrace. Understanding that these sentiments are ordinary is the most vital move towards tending to them. Recognizing and communicating feelings can be freeing and enabling, permitting people to deal with their sentiments and push ahead.

Emotionally supportive networks assume a vital part in the profound excursion. Friends and family, companions, and care groups give priceless comprehension and solace during attempting times. Medical services experts likewise offer consistent reassurance, directing people through the intricacies of analysis, therapy choices, and recuperation.

Besides, looking for information and data is an integral asset for profound versatility. Grasping the condition, its treatment choices, and the potential results can reduce nervousness and vulnerability. Information is a wellspring of strengthening and a method for assuming command of one's medical services venture.

The close to home excursion is a huge part of the HPV experience. By recognizing and tending to these sentiments, looking for help, and remaining informed, people can transcend the personal difficulties presented by HPV and its related medical problems. This section fills in as a directing light through this piece of the excursion, offering bits of knowledge and consolation to assist people with exploring their profound way and arise more grounded on the opposite side.

Adapting to a HPV Determination

Getting a HPV determination can be a sincerely difficult encounter. This part digs into the systems and contemplations for adapting to a HPV conclusion, offering experiences on how people can explore the profound and down to earth parts of this life changing second.

Quite possibly the earliest and most significant advances is recognizing and handling the feelings that accompany a HPV conclusion. Dread, disarray, and nervousness are normal responses. It's fundamental to comprehend that these feelings are completely typical and that contacting friends and family or an encouraging group of people can give truly necessary solace and understanding.

Looking for precise data is another fundamental way of dealing with especially difficult times. Grasping the sort of HPV, its possible dangers, and the accessible medicines is engaging. Information can disperse vulnerabilities and assist people with arriving at informed conclusions about their medical care venture.

Keeping up with open correspondence with medical care experts is pivotal. They can direct people through the finding, make sense of the ramifications, and suggest fitting medicines or observing. Participating in fair conversations about the condition and the accessible choices can offer consolation and backing.

Adapting to a HPV determination frequently includes flexibility and profound strength. An extraordinary excursion can prompt self-awareness and strengthening. By tending to feelings, looking for information, and remaining associated with medical care suppliers and encouraging groups of people, people can explore this difficult second and set up for their way towards recuperation and prosperity. This section fills in as a guide for people confronting a HPV determination, offering direction and bits of knowledge on the most proficient method to adapt and arise more grounded from this life changing experience.

Building Areas of strength for an Organization

Despite a HPV finding and its connected difficulties, having major areas of strength for an organization resembles a wellbeing net, giving solace, understanding, and direction. This section highlights the meaning of building and keeping a vigorous encouraging group of people and offers experiences into how to develop one during troublesome times.

Loved ones are in many cases the principal line of help. Their affection, empathy, and presence can offer vast solace. Discussing your thoughts and worries with those near you can give a close to home delivery and make a feeling of satisfaction.

Medical services experts assume a basic part in your encouraging group of people. They give clinical direction as well as basic encouragement. Building a trusting and open relationship with your medical care group permits you to clarify some pressing issues, look for explanation, and examine your interests, encouraging a feeling that everything is good during your medical care venture.

Support gatherings, whether face to face or on the web, offer an extraordinary type of understanding. Interfacing with other people who are going through comparative encounters can make a feeling of kinship and the consolation that you're in good company in your excursion.

In addition, emotional wellness experts can offer important help for close to home prosperity. They are gifted at assisting people with handling their sentiments and foster survival methods for managing pressure and nervousness.

Building serious areas of strength for an organization is a proactive move toward dealing with a HPV finding and its inner difficulties. The consolidated strength of family, companions, medical care experts, support gatherings, and psychological wellness specialists makes a strong starting point for profound flexibility and a conviction that all is good during troublesome times. This part fills in as a manual for help people sustain and keep up with their encouraging groups of people as they explore the intricacies of HPV-related medical problems.

Embracing Life Beyond the Diagnosis

An HPV diagnosis may feel like a life-altering event, but it doesn't define you. This chapter delves into the journey of embracing life beyond the diagnosis, highlighting the possibilities of resilience, personal growth, and renewed hope.

The first step in moving forward is to acknowledge the diagnosis as a part of your journey, not the entirety of it. Understanding that an HPV diagnosis is a medical condition, not a life sentence, allows you to retain a sense of identity beyond the virus.

Setting realistic goals for yourself is another essential aspect of post-diagnosis life. Focusing on your well-being, both physical and emotional, and pursuing the things that bring you joy and purpose can help you regain control of your life.

It's crucial to remember that an HPV diagnosis doesn't mean you're alone. Lean on your support network for encouragement and seek guidance from healthcare professionals. They can offer insights on your treatment options and your journey to recovery.

Furthermore, consider becoming an advocate for HPV awareness and prevention. Sharing your experiences can help reduce the stigma surrounding the virus and empower others to take control of their health through vaccination and regular screenings.

Embracing life beyond the diagnosis is a journey of healing, resilience, and personal growth. By acknowledging the diagnosis as part of your life story, setting goals, seeking support, and advocating for HPV awareness, you can create a new chapter filled with hope, empowerment, and a renewed zest for life.

CHAPTER EIGHT

Beyond the Individual: Supporting Caregivers

In the context of Human Papilloma virus (HPV) and its associated health issues, it's essential to recognize that caregivers also play a significant role in the healthcare journey. This chapter highlights the importance of supporting caregivers and offers insights into how to assist and acknowledge their vital contributions.

Caregivers, often family members or close friends, are on the frontline of support for individuals dealing with HPV-related health issues. They provide emotional support, help with daily activities, and act as advocates within the healthcare system. Their role is pivotal in ensuring the well-being and recovery of those affected.

Recognizing the toll that caregiving can take, it's vital to provide caregivers with the support they need. Encourage them to seek their own support networks, as they can also benefit from sharing experiences and receiving guidance. This will help them manage the emotional and physical challenges that come with caregiving.

Offering respite care, allowing caregivers to take a break and recharge, can be a valuable form of support. It acknowledges the sacrifices they make and prevents caregiver burnout.

Furthermore, including caregivers in healthcare discussions and decisions is critical. They can provide invaluable insights into the patient's well-being and preferences, contributing to a more comprehensive approach to care.

Supporting caregivers is a vital component of the healthcare journey. This chapter shines a light on their contributions and the importance of providing them with the support they need. By acknowledging and aiding caregivers, we ensure a more holistic and compassionate approach to managing HPV-related health issues, promoting the well-being of both patients and their dedicated caregivers.

A Helping Hand for Partners and Caregivers

Partners and caregivers are often the unsung heroes in the journey of individuals facing HPV-related health challenges. This chapter underscores the significance of offering a helping hand to these dedicated individuals and provides insights into how they can navigate the complexities of their roles with compassion and support.

Partners of individuals dealing with HPV-related health issues often play a pivotal role in providing emotional support. They can be a pillar of strength, offering understanding and comfort during difficult times. Engaging in open and empathetic communication can foster a sense of trust and solidarity within the relationship.

For caregivers, often family members or close friends, the journey can be physically and emotionally demanding. Offering respite care and encouraging self-care are essential. Caregivers must also recognize their own limits and seek support networks to help them manage the challenges they face.

In both roles, education is a powerful tool. Partners and caregivers can seek information about HPV, its associated health risks, and the available treatments. This knowledge allows them to provide more informed support and be better prepared to assist individuals through their healthcare journey.

The chapter highlights the significance of offering a helping hand to partners and caregivers, recognizing their essential roles in providing emotional, physical, and practical support. By understanding and addressing their needs, we create a more compassionate and comprehensive approach to managing HPV-related health issues, supporting not only the individuals affected but also those who stand by them in their journey.

How to Provide Emotional Support

Emotional support is often the cornerstone of helping individuals dealing with HPV-related health issues to navigate their journey with resilience and hope. This chapter offers insights into how to provide this essential support with understanding and compassion.

First and foremost, active listening is a powerful tool for emotional support. Encourage open and honest communication, and be a non-judgmental and empathetic presence. Allow the individual to express their feelings, concerns, and fears without interruption.

Validation is equally important. Acknowledge the person's emotions and experiences as real and significant. It's crucial to let them know that their feelings are entirely normal and that they are not alone in their journey.

Offering encouragement and positivity can also be a source of comfort. Provide reassurance and remind the individual of their strengths and resilience. Celebrate their successes, no matter how small, and share in their hope for the future.

Creating a safe and understanding environment is essential. Give the person space to express their emotions and concerns without feeling pressured to "move on" or "get over it."

Patience is key, as emotional healing is a process that varies for each individual.

Finally, consider suggesting professional help when necessary. Mental health professionals can provide valuable guidance in processing emotions and developing effective coping strategies.

Providing emotional support is an act of empathy, compassion, and understanding. By following these guidelines, you can be a pillar of strength for individuals navigating HPV-related health issues, helping them to find solace, hope, and a sense of control in their journey.

Strengthening Relationships Through Understanding

The journey through HPV-related health issues can place a considerable strain on relationships, but it can also be an opportunity to deepen understanding and strengthen bonds.

This chapter explores how couples and families can navigate these challenges, fostering empathy, support, and resilience.

Effective communication is a cornerstone of understanding within relationships. Open and honest discussions can help partners share their feelings, fears, and hopes. It's important to create a safe space for both individuals to express their emotions and concerns without judgment.

Empathy is another crucial aspect. Partners can strive to understand each other's perspectives and experiences, acknowledging that everyone processes difficult situations differently. This shared empathy can create a strong foundation for mutual support.

Moreover, engaging in education together can deepen understanding. Learning about HPV, its potential risks, and the available treatments can empower couples to make informed decisions and tackle the challenges as a united front.

Offering practical support can also strengthen relationships. Whether it's attending medical appointments together, assisting with daily tasks, or providing emotional comfort, these acts of support show care and love during difficult times.

The chapter highlights that, while HPV-related health issues may present challenges, they also present an opportunity for growth and deeper connection within relationships. By fostering understanding, communication, and support, couples and families can navigate these challenges with resilience and emerge even stronger on the other side.

CHAPTER NINE

Your Health, Your Responsibility: Staying Informed

Getting a sense of ownership with your wellbeing is a major part of overseeing HPV-related medical problems really. This section highlights the significance of remaining educated and participated in your medical services excursion to pursue informed choices, advocate for yourself, and keep a feeling of control.

Remaining informed starts with looking for precise data about HPV, its related wellbeing gambles, and the accessible counteraction and treatment choices. Schooling enables you to comprehend your condition, settle on informed decisions, and effectively take part in your medical care choices.

Routine screenings are an essential piece of remaining informed. Customary check-ups, including Pap spreads and HPV tests, are fundamental for early recognition and mediation. By remaining current with these screenings, you can screen your wellbeing and address any worries speedily.

Powerful correspondence with medical care experts is critical. Clarify some pressing issues, look for explanation, and take part in open conversations about your condition, treatment choices, and any worries or aftereffects. Coordinated effort with your medical care group guarantees that your remarkable necessities and inclinations are thought of.

Embracing a proactive way to deal with your wellbeing incorporates way of life decisions, for example, taking on a reasonable eating regimen, keeping up with actual work, and keeping away from tobacco and over the top liquor utilization. These decisions add to in general prosperity and lessen the gamble of HPV-related sicknesses.

Your wellbeing is for sure your obligation. By remaining educated, partaking effectively in your medical services choices, and embracing a preventive way to deal with prosperity, you can assume command over your excursion through HPV-related medical problems. This section fills in as a manual for assist you with exploring this way with information and certainty, at last guaranteeing the most ideal results for your wellbeing.

Focusing on Standard Check-ups and Screenings

Standard check-ups and screenings are foundations of keeping up with your wellbeing, particularly with regards to HPV-related medical problems. This part underscores the meaning of focusing on these arrangements and offers experiences into how they assume a vital part in early location and counteraction.

Standard check-ups act as proactive measures in protecting your wellbeing. They permit medical services experts to screen your prosperity, spot early admonition signs, and intercede before medical problems raise. Focusing on these arrangements guarantees that your wellbeing is reliably observed and any worries are tended to speedily.

Screenings, for example, Pap spreads and HPV tests, are explicit apparatuses for early discovery of HPV-related conditions. These tests can distinguish cell changes or the presence of the infection, taking into account mediation before potential medical problems create. Focusing on standard screenings is a proactive move toward forestalling the movement of HPV-related sicknesses.

Understanding the significance of screenings and check-ups with regards to HPV is fundamental. High-risk HPV strains can frequently stay asymptomatic, making early identification critical. Obligation to these arrangements safeguards your wellbeing as well as adds to general wellbeing by decreasing the transmission of the infection.

This section fills in as a sign of the obligation you have for your wellbeing. Focusing on customary check-ups and screenings is an interest in your prosperity and a proactive measure to forestall and identify HPV-related medical problems early. By remaining focused on these arrangements, you assume command over your wellbeing and guarantee that potential worries are tended to instantly, prompting a better and safer future.

Remaining Informed for a Long period of Wellbeing

Wellbeing isn't an objective; it's a long lasting excursion. This section accentuates the benefit of remaining educated and participated in your wellbeing all through your lifetime, especially with regards to HPV-related medical problems. It offers experiences into how predictable carefulness can prompt better wellbeing results and a greater of life.

Long lasting wellbeing starts with a pledge to grasping your wellbeing. Consistent training and remaining informed about HPV, its expected dangers, and the significance of avoidance is vital. By learning and remaining refreshed, you enable yourself to pursue informed choices and promoter for your prosperity.

Consistency in standard check-ups and screenings is one more imperative part of deep rooted health. HPV and its connected medical problems can influence people at different life stages, making normal screenings pivotal. By keeping up with this responsibility all through your life, you guarantee that any worries are identified and tended to speedily.

Way of life decisions, for example, rehearsing safe sex, keeping a reasonable eating routine, remaining truly dynamic, and keeping away from tobacco and exorbitant liquor utilization, likewise assume a critical part in long lasting wellbeing. These decisions add to your general wellbeing and decrease the gamble of HPV-related infections.

This section fills in as an update that remaining educated and participated in your wellbeing is a promise to a long period of health. By getting a sense of ownership with your prosperity, reliably looking for training and screenings, and settling on sound way of life decisions, you upgrade your personal satisfaction and guarantee a better and safer future for yourself.

The Force of Information: How You Can Have an Effect

In the domain of Human Papilloma infection (HPV) and its connected medical problems, information is a powerful device that can change lives and have a tremendous effect. This part highlights the groundbreaking force of information and offers bits of knowledge into how people can utilize it to make positive change.

Figuring out HPV, its transmission, counteraction, and potential dangers is the most vital phase in having an effect. With this information, you can turn into a proactive supporter for you and others, bringing issues to light and cultivating counteraction.

Sharing data is a vital method for having an effect. By teaching companions, family, and your local area about the significance of HPV inoculations, customary screenings, and safe sex rehearses, you add to an aggregate work to diminish the weight of HPV-related sicknesses.

Supporting approach change is one more road for influence. You can advocate for further developed admittance to inoculations and screenings, assisting with guaranteeing that medical care assets are accessible to all. Drawing in with policymakers and partaking in general wellbeing drives enhances your impact in the battle against HPV.

Partaking in research and clinical preliminaries is a more straightforward method for having an effect. Your inclusion adds to the improvement of new medicines and anticipation methodologies, propelling the field of HPV research.

This section fills in as an update that information is an impetus for change. By grasping HPV and its suggestions and finding a way proactive ways to teach, advocate, support strategy change, and take part in research, you saddle the force of information to have a massive effect in the fight against HPV-related medical problems, eventually adding to a better future for all.

CHAPTER TEN

Empowering Tomorrow: The Call to Action

The fight against Human Papilloma infection (HPV) and its related medical problems is an aggregate exertion that calls for activity and responsibility. This part fills in as a revitalizing cry to move people, networks, and society all in all to take a proactive position in this fight.

Strengthening starts with information. Figuring out the dangers of HPV and the significance of vaccinations, standard screenings, and safe sex rehearses is the underpinning of activity. By remaining educated and instructed, people can safeguard themselves and backer for those they care about.

Bringing issues to light is a basic source of inspiration. By sharing data about HPV, scattering legends and misinterpretations, and advancing inoculation and early identification, you can add to a culture of wellbeing and counteraction. Mindfulness crusades, local area occasions, and instructive drives can assume a vital part in this work.

Support for strategy change is another fundamental stage. People can draw in with administrators and general wellbeing foundations to guarantee that assets are coordinated toward HPV counteraction, examination, and admittance to medical care administrations.

Cooperation in research and clinical preliminaries promotes the battle against HPV-related medical problems. By chipping in for examinations, you can straightforwardly affect the improvement of new therapies and anticipation methodologies, pushing the limits of clinical science.

Enabling tomorrow isn't simply a source of inspiration; it's a guarantee to a better, more secure future for all. By taking a proactive position, remaining educated, bringing issues to light, supporting for strategy change, and partaking in examination, people and networks can drive change and have a massive effect in the fight against HPV-related medical problems.

Rundown of Fundamental Focus points

In the excursion through the intricacies of Human Papilloma infection (HPV) and its related medical problems, a few pivotal focal points arise as core values for people and networks. This rundown typifies the vital examples and fundamental experiences from the book, giving a guide to exploring the difficulties of HPV and advancing a future liberated from its weights.

1. Knowledge is Empowerment: Grasping HPV, its transmission, and counteraction is the primary line of guard. Schooling enables people to pursue informed choices, advocate for their wellbeing, and add to HPV mindfulness.

2. Early Location Saves Lives: Standard check-ups and screenings, for example, Pap spreads and HPV tests, are imperative for early discovery and intercession. Focusing on these arrangements can forestall the movement of HPV-related illnesses.

3. Support Organizations Matter: Building solid encouraging groups of people, including family, companions, medical care experts, and care groups, is fundamental. Basic reassurance and understanding are essential during testing times.

4. Wellness is a Deep rooted Journey: Long lasting wellbeing expects obligation to schooling, counteraction, and a reasonable way of life. Remaining educated and proactive about your wellbeing is fundamental at each life stage.

5. Advocacy Makes Change: Upholding for HPV mindfulness and strategy change intensifies the effect on a local area and cultural level. Association in research and clinical preliminaries adds to logical headways.

6. Empathy Reinforces Relationships: Sympathy, open correspondence, and common help inside connections can assist people and their accomplices with exploring the profound and reasonable difficulties of HPV-related medical problems.

7. Hope and Resilience: Survivors' accounts and the force of flexibility highlight the potential for development and individual strength even with HPV-related medical problems.

8. Supporting Caregivers: Recognizing and offering help for parental figures is essentially as critical as supporting those straightforwardly impacted by HPV. Perceive their commitments and proposition help when required.

9. A Long lasting Commitment: Deep rooted wellbeing includes continuous check-ups, schooling, and way of life decisions. Getting a sense of ownership with your wellbeing guarantees a better, safer future.

10. Your Job in the Battle: Individual activities can have a tremendous effect in the fight against HPV. By remaining informed, upholding for counteraction, and partaking in research, you add to a better future for all.

These fundamental focus points act as a directing light for people and networks, stressing the significance of information, counteraction, backing, and support in the battle against HPV-related medical problems. By embracing these standards, we can by and large have an effect and work towards a future liberated from the weights of HPV.

Joining the HPV Awareness Movement

Joining the HPV awareness movement is an invitation to be part of a global initiative that seeks to educate, advocate, and eradicate the impact of Human Papilloma virus (HPV) on individuals and communities. This chapter delves into the importance of becoming an active participant in this movement, highlighting how your involvement can make a meaningful difference.

At the heart of the awareness movement is education. By taking part, you become an informed advocate, capable of dispelling myths and misconceptions about HPV. Your knowledge becomes a beacon of light, guiding those around you toward the path of prevention and early detection.

Advocacy is another cornerstone of this movement. Your voice can influence policy changes, improved access to vaccinations and screenings, and increased support for HPV research. By participating in advocacy efforts, you contribute to a societal shift towards a culture of health and prevention.

Sharing your own story can be a powerful tool in raising awareness. Your experiences can provide a sense of connection and hope for those going through similar challenges. Your courage in sharing your journey can inspire and empower others.

Finally, participating in community events, awareness campaigns, and educational initiatives amplifies your impact. By joining forces with like-minded individuals and organizations, you can create a wave of change that ripples across communities and beyond.

Joining the HPV awareness movement is not just an invitation; it's a call to action. By becoming an active participant, you empower yourself and others to take control of their health and contribute to a future free from the burdens of HPV. Your involvement can create lasting change, offering hope and a healthier future for all.

CHAPTER ELEVEN

Becoming a Part of the Solution

In the battle against Human Papilloma virus (HPV) and its associated health issues, becoming a part of the solution is an impactful and empowering choice. This chapter emphasizes the role that each individual can play in creating a positive change and outlines the steps to actively contribute to this cause.

Education is the first step toward becoming a part of the solution. Understanding HPV, its transmission, prevention, and associated risks equips you with the knowledge necessary to make informed decisions and share critical information with others.

Advocacy is another crucial component. By becoming a vocal advocate for HPV awareness, you can influence policy changes and garner support for increased access to vaccinations, screenings, and research funding. Your voice is a catalyst for change in your community and on a broader scale.

Participating in research and clinical trials is a more direct way to contribute to the solution. Your involvement can advance medical science, leading to the development of improved treatments and prevention strategies.

Raising awareness is a powerful tool in your arsenal. By sharing your knowledge and experiences with friends, family, and your community, you can help dispel misconceptions and foster a culture of health and prevention.

This chapter serves as an invitation to individuals to actively participate in the solution to HPV-related health issues. By educating themselves, advocating for change, participating in research, and raising awareness, they can make a significant impact and contribute to a future free from the burdens of HPV.

A Treasure Trove of Reputable Sources

The quest for reliable information in the realm of Human Papilloma virus (HPV) and its related health issues is vital to making informed decisions and taking charge of one's well-being. This section is a treasure trove of reputable sources that individuals can explore for a deeper understanding of HPV and its implications.

1. Centers for Disease Control and Prevention (CDC): The CDC is a gold standard for information on public health. Their website provides comprehensive resources on HPV, including vaccination guidelines and factsheets.

2. World Health Organization (WHO): As a global health authority, WHO offers in-depth reports and information about HPV's worldwide impact, prevention strategies, and global health policies.

3. National Cancer Institute (NCI): NCI offers extensive research and information on HPV's role in cancer, providing valuable insights into the links between HPV and specific cancers.

4. American Cancer Society: This organization provides resources on HPV-related cancers, screening guidelines, and treatment options, offering a wealth of information and support for patients and their families.

5. American Sexual Health Association (ASHA): ASHA is a reputable source for sexual health information, including HPV, offering guidance, educational materials, and support.

6. International Papillomavirus Society (IPVS): This society focuses on advancing the scientific and medical understanding of HPV. Their website offers resources on research, prevention, and treatment.

7. Medical Journals: Leading medical journals such as "The Lancet" and "Vaccine" regularly publish research studies, clinical trials, and reviews on HPV and its vaccines, providing cutting-edge information.

8. Government Healthcare Websites: National and local government healthcare websites often offer guidelines,

vaccination programs, and information on where to get vaccinated.

These reputable sources serve as valuable guides for those seeking to expand their knowledge and make informed decisions regarding HPV and related health issues. By delving into these sources, individuals can empower themselves with reliable information and take proactive steps towards prevention, early detection, and overall well-being.

Dive Deeper into the World of HPV

The world of Human Papilloma virus (HPV) is complex, with its implications spanning from cervical cancer to genital warts and more. To fully grasp its impact, one can dive deeper into this realm, uncovering both its medical and societal dimensions. This section invites individuals to explore the multifaceted facets of HPV, deepening their understanding and awareness.

Medical Insights: Understanding the medical aspects of HPV is crucial. Delve into the different types and strains of HPV, their modes of transmission, and the potential health risks they pose. Learn about the science of HPV vaccines, screening methods, and treatment options for HPV-related conditions.

Prevention and Vaccination:Explore the world of HPV prevention. Learn about the importance of HPV vaccinations and their impact on reducing the prevalence of HPV-related diseases. Dive into the vaccination guidelines, benefits, and potential side effects to make informed decisions.

Personal Stories: HPV isn't just a medical condition; it affects real people. Read personal stories and experiences of individuals who have faced HPV-related challenges. These narratives shed light on the emotional and practical aspects of living with and overcoming HPV.

Global Impact: Discover the global impact of HPV and the efforts being made to combat it on a global scale. Investigate organizations, initiatives, and international policies aimed at reducing the burden of HPV-related diseases.

Community Involvement: Dive into the world of HPV awareness and advocacy. Explore how you can become an active participant in the HPV awareness movement, sharing information, raising awareness, and advocating for policy changes that benefit public health.

By delving deeper into the world of HPV, individuals can gain a more comprehensive understanding of this virus and its far-reaching effects. This knowledge equips them to make informed choices, contribute to the prevention of HPV-related diseases, and become agents of change in their communities and the world at large.

Additional Reading for the Curious Mind

For those with a curious mind eager to explore the complexities of Human Papilloma virus (HPV) and its related health issues, an array of engaging and insightful books can serve as invaluable resources. This section presents a selection of additional reading recommendations that cater to various interests and aspects of

HPV, from scientific research to personal narratives and public health perspectives.

1. The HPV Vaccine Controversy: Sex, Cancer, God, and Politics by Anna Kirkland: This book delves into the cultural, political, and medical aspects of the HPV vaccine, shedding light on the controversies surrounding it.

2. Cancer, HPV, and Me: 20 Years Later by Will Cochrane: A personal account of the author's journey with HPV-related cancer, offering insights into the emotional and practical aspects of living with and overcoming the condition.

3. The Coming Plague: Newly Emerging Diseases in a World Out of Balance by Laurie Garrett: While not solely focused on HPV, this book provides a broader perspective on emerging diseases and their global impact.

4. The Immortal Life of Henrietta Lacks by Rebecca Skloot: A remarkable true story that touches on medical ethics, informed consent, and the use of human cells in scientific research, providing a unique perspective on medical advancements, including those related to HPV.

5. Gulp: Adventures on the Alimentary Canal by Mary Roach: Though not exclusively about HPV, this book explores various aspects of the human body, including its interactions with viruses and diseases, offering a lighthearted and curious perspective on science and health.

6. The Emperor of All Maladies: A Biography of Cancer by Siddhartha Mukherjee: While focusing on cancer, this book explores the history, science, and personal stories related to the disease, which has overlapping implications with HPV-related cancers.

These books offer an array of perspectives on HPV and its associated health issues, catering to the inquisitive reader interested in scientific research, personal narratives, public health discussions, and more. Exploring these texts can provide a well-rounded understanding of the multifaceted world of HPV, from its scientific underpinnings to its emotional and societal dimensions.

CONCLUSION

Your Journey of Empowerment

Your journey through the complexities of Human Papilloma virus (HPV) and its associated health issues is not just a path of challenges; it is also a journey of empowerment. This section celebrates your empowerment as you navigate the world of HPV, offering insights into how you can assert control over your health, make informed decisions, and inspire others to do the same.

Knowledge as Power: Education is the cornerstone of your empowerment. By understanding HPV, its transmission, prevention, and related health risks, you become an informed advocate. Your knowledge is a shield against misinformation and a weapon against the virus.

Advocacy and Awareness: Your voice has the power to change lives. By advocating for HPV awareness, you influence public health policies, increase access to vaccinations and screenings, and promote a culture of prevention. Your advocacy can save lives.

Survivor Stories: Personal stories, including your own, are a source of inspiration. By sharing your experiences and triumphs over HPV-related challenges, you offer hope and strength to others who may be facing similar situations. Your story can be a guiding light.

Support Networks: Your journey is not solitary. Friends, family, healthcare professionals, and support groups provide a network of emotional and practical support. By seeking and utilizing these resources, you strengthen your resilience.

A Future of Wellness: Ultimately, your journey is a pursuit of wellness. By taking control of your health, participating in screenings, making informed choices, and embracing a proactive approach, you pave the way for a healthier future.

Your journey through HPV is a path of empowerment, and your actions have the potential to change lives. By wielding the power of knowledge, advocacy, personal stories, support networks, and a commitment to wellness, you not only empower yourself but also inspire those around you to take charge of their health. Your journey becomes a beacon of hope and an example of resilience for others to follow.

Reminding You That Knowledge Is Your Best Ally

In the intricate landscape of Human Papilloma virus (HPV) and its associated health issues, knowledge stands as your most reliable and steadfast ally. This section serves as a reminder of the profound significance of knowledge in your journey, underlining how it equips you to navigate challenges, make informed decisions, and embrace a proactive stance toward your health.

Understanding HPV: Knowledge of HPV, from its transmission to the potential risks it poses, empowers you with the information necessary to make informed choices about prevention, treatment, and lifestyle.

Prevention and Vaccination: Awareness of the available HPV vaccines and their benefits enables you to take proactive measures to protect yourself and others from HPV-related health issues.

Early Detection and Screening: Knowledge of screening methods and their importance in early detection empowers you to stay ahead of potential health concerns and seek timely medical intervention.

Advocacy and Awareness: Equipped with knowledge, you can become a vocal advocate for HPV awareness, influencing policy changes, and dispelling myths and misconceptions that may hinder public health efforts.

Emotional Resilience: Understanding the emotional and practical aspects of living with HPV-related health issues provides you with a sense of preparedness and emotional resilience.

As you traverse the complexities of HPV, always remember that knowledge is your steadfast companion. It guides your decisions, equips you to advocate for yourself and others, and contributes to a culture of prevention. Knowledge empowers you to take control of your health, ultimately ensuring a healthier and more secure future.